TABLE OF CONTENTS

PREFACE

Prepare to be astounded as you delve into the harrowing journey of Noah, an ordinary man whose life was turned upside down by the unprecedented COVID-19 pandemic. This is not just another pandemic story; this is a raw, unfiltered look into the depths of human resilience and the fragility of the mind. Uncover the shocking truth behind one man's descent into madness, a chilling testament to the mental toll of the global crisis.

This unbelievable story will leave you speechless, as you navigate through the highs and lows of Noah's life pre and post the pandemic's arrival. From the calm before the storm to the heart-wrenching struggle with isolation and despair, you'll be on the edge of your seat, gripped by the stark reality of his experiences. This is a tale that will make you question everything you thought you knew about mental health.

Noah's story is a stark reminder of the unseen battles many are fighting in the wake of the pandemic. It's a wake-up call for society to acknowledge and address the mental health crisis that has been exacerbated by the pandemic. As you turn the pages of 'From Sanity to Madness: How the Pandemic Pushed One Man to the Edge of Insanity!', prepare to have your perceptions challenged, your emotions stirred, and your understanding of mental health during a pandemic forever changed.

INTRODUCTION: THE CALM BEFORE THE STORM

In Fort Myers, FL where life moved at a leisurely pace and everyone knew everyone, Noah Thompson was a familiar face. A high school teacher by profession, he was known for his infectious enthusiasm and his ability to make even the most complex concepts seem simple. Outside the classroom, he was a loving husband, a doting father, and an avid reader with a penchant for cooking. His life was a harmonious blend of work, family, and hobbies, a life that was about to be disrupted by an unforeseen storm.

As 2019 drew to a close, Noah, like the rest of the world, was looking forward to the new year with optimism and hope. He had plans, dreams, and aspirations, all of which seemed within reach. But as the saying goes, "Man proposes, God disposes." The year 2020 had other plans, plans that would challenge Noah's resilience and strength, plans that would push him to the brink of his sanity.

In the early days of 2020, news of a novel virus started making the rounds. It was a distant problem, something that was happening in another part of the world. It was something that was reported on the news, but it didn't seem to have any direct impact on Noah's day-to-day life. He went about his routine, unaware of the storm that was brewing halfway across the world.

As the days turned into weeks, the news of the virus became more frequent and more alarming. It was no longer confined to a distant land; it was spreading, crossing borders and oceans, inching closer to Florida with each passing day. The virus, now known as COVID-19, was no longer a distant problem; it was a looming threat.

Noah, like everyone else, watched the news with a growing sense of unease. He saw the numbers of infected and deceased rising, the healthcare systems of powerful nations crumbling under the strain, and the fear and panic that was gripping the world. He saw the world changing, and he knew that his life, too, was about to change.

As the first case of COVID-19 was reported in Florida, the state went into lockdown. Schools were closed, businesses were shuttered, and the once bustling streets were eerily quiet. Noah found himself confined to his home, grappling with the new reality of remote teaching, worrying about the safety of his family, and trying to make sense of the chaos that was unfolding around him.

As I continue to share the story of Noah, I invite you, dear readers, to keep reading and discover the journey that unfolds before us.

CHAPTER 1: A NORMAL LIFE PRE-PANDEMIC

Once upon a time, in a world that seemed familiar yet suddenly turned upside down, there lived a man named Noah Thompson. Before the world was gripped by the pandemic, Noah led a life that was as ordinary as it was fulfilling. He was a man of simple pleasures, finding joy in the everyday routine that many took for granted. His life was a tapestry of work, family, friends, and hobbies, each thread intertwining to create a picture of contentment and balance.

Noah worked as a high school teacher in Fort Myers, FL. He was passionate about his job, finding immense satisfaction in shaping young minds and preparing them for the future. His students admired him, not just for his knowledge and teaching skills, but also for his ability to connect with them on a personal level. He was more than just a teacher; he was a mentor, a guide, and a friend.

Outside of work, Noah was a family man. He was a devoted husband to his wife, Emily, and a doting father to their two children, Lily and Max. Family time was sacred to Noah. Whether it was helping with homework, playing in the backyard, or simply enjoying a quiet dinner together, these moments were the highlights of his day.

Noah also had a close-knit group of friends. They had known each other since college and had managed to stay connected despite the demands of work and family. They met regularly, their gatherings filled with laughter, reminiscing, and friendly banter. These friendships were a source of comfort and support for Noah, a reminder of the bond they shared.

In his spare time, Noah loved to read. He had an extensive collection of books, ranging from classic literature to contemporary fiction. Reading was his escape, a way to unwind and lose himself in different worlds and stories. He also had a penchant for cooking. He found it therapeutic, a creative outlet that allowed him to experiment with flavors and create delicious meals for his family. His Sunday roasts were legendary, eagerly anticipated by his family and friends.

Noah was also an active member of his community. He volunteered at the local food bank, coached the neighborhood kids' soccer team, and was always ready to lend a helping hand. His kindness and generosity were well-known, earning him the respect and admiration of those around him.

His life was a delicate balance of work, family, friends, and personal interests. It was a life filled with love, laughter, and fulfillment. It was a life that was about to be disrupted by an unforeseen force.

He continued his daily routine - teaching his students, spending time with his family, meeting his friends, and volunteering in his community. Life went on as usual, but there was a growing sense of unease, a feeling of impending doom that was hard to shake off.

The virus, now named COVID-19, was declared a pandemic by the World Health Organization. The news sent shockwaves around the world. Everything was closed, and people were advised to stay at home. The world as Noah knew it was changing, and it was changing fast.

Noah found himself in a new reality, a reality where he was confined to his home, where he couldn't go to work or meet his friends, where his children couldn't go to school, where the simple act of stepping outside was fraught with fear and anxiety. It was a reality that was far removed from the normalcy and routine he was accustomed to.

As he grappled with this new reality, Noah couldn't help but long for his pre-pandemic life. He missed his students, his friends, and his community. He missed the hustle and bustle of his everyday life, the simple pleasures he had taken for granted. He missed the freedom, the spontaneity, the predictability of his old life.

His home, once a place of comfort and joy, now felt like a prison. His days, once filled with meaningful interactions and activities, now seemed empty and monotonous. His mind, once occupied with lesson plans and family outings, was now consumed with worry and fear.

Despite the challenges, Noah tried to maintain a sense of normalcy. He started teaching his students online, a new experience that was both challenging and rewarding. He spent more time with his family, cherishing the moments of togetherness amidst the uncertainty. He stayed connected with his friends through video calls, their virtual gatherings a source of comfort and solace.

He also found solace in his hobbies. He read more, losing himself in the pages of his books. He cooked more, experimenting with new recipes and flavors. These activities, though simple, provided a much-needed distraction from the grim reality of the pandemic.

Yet, despite his best efforts, Noah couldn't shake off the feeling of unease.

CHAPTER 2: THE ARRIVAL OF THE PANDEMIC

The calm before the storm had passed, and Noah was now in the eye of the pandemic storm. His life, like the lives of millions around the world, was turned upside down. But amidst the fear and uncertainty, Noah found a strength he didn't know he possessed. He found the courage to face the storm, to adapt to the new normal, and to keep going, one day at a time.

As the world battled the pandemic, Noah battled his own storm. He faced the challenges with determination and resilience, proving that even in the darkest of times, the human spirit can shine bright. This is the story of Noah, a story of courage, resilience, and hope in the face of a global pandemic.

Noah Thompson, like everyone else, watched the unfolding crisis with a growing sense of dread. He had seen the news reports from other countries, the overwhelmed hospitals, the rising death toll, the fear and panic. He had hoped, prayed even, that Florida would be spared. But the virus, it seemed, was indiscriminate.

The school where Noah taught was one of the first institutions to close its doors. The announcement came on a Friday, a sudden end to the normalcy of school life. Noah found himself packing up his classroom, a strange sense of finality hanging in the air. As he locked the door behind him, he couldn't help but wonder when he would be back, when things would return to normal.

But normal, as Noah soon discovered, was a thing of the past. The town went into lockdown, a necessary measure to slow the spread of the virus. The streets, once filled with the sounds of everyday life, fell silent. Businesses closed, events were canceled, and people retreated into their homes, their lives put on hold.

Noah's home became his sanctuary, his classroom, his world. He set up a makeshift classroom in his study, adapting to the new reality of remote teaching. It was a challenge, to say the least. The lively discussions, the hands-on experiments, the lightbulb moments - all were lost in the transition to online learning. But Noah persevered, determined to provide his students with a sense of normalcy amidst the chaos. He spent hours preparing lessons, recording videos, and answering emails, trying to bridge the gap created by the physical distance.

At the same time, Noah grappled with the fear and uncertainty that the pandemic brought. He worried about his family, their health, and their safety. His wife, a nurse at the local hospital, was on the front lines of the battle against the virus. Each day, she left for work with a brave smile, but Noah could see the worry in her eyes. Their two children, too young to fully understand the gravity of the situation, looked to their parents for reassurance and comfort.

The pandemic also brought with it a sense of isolation. Noah missed the camaraderie of his colleagues, the chatter of his students, and the simple pleasure of a shared meal with friends. The days seemed to blend into each other, each one a repetition of the one before. The world outside his window seemed to have come to a standstill, a stark contrast to the turmoil inside his mind.

Yet, amidst the fear and uncertainty, Noah found moments of hope and resilience. He found it in the way his community came together, supporting each other in these trying times. He found it in the laughter of his children, a reminder of the joy and innocence that still existed in the world. He found it in the quiet moments with his wife, their bond strengthening in the face of adversity. He found it in his students, their eagerness to learn undiminished by the circumstances.

Noah also found solace in his hobbies. He spent his free time reading, losing himself in the pages of books, finding comfort in the familiar rhythm of words. He experimented with new recipes, the act of cooking serving as a therapeutic escape from the harsh reality outside.

The arrival of the pandemic was a test of Noah's resilience. It pushed him to his limits, challenging him in ways he had never imagined. But it also revealed a strength he didn't know he possessed. He learned to adapt, to persevere, to find hope in the darkest of times.

As the days turned into weeks, and the weeks into months, Noah held on to that hope. He held on to the belief that this storm, too, would pass. That they would emerge from it stronger and more resilient. That they would find their way back to normal, a new normal perhaps, but a normal, nonetheless.

The pandemic was a storm that had disrupted Noah's life, but it was also a storm that had shown him what truly mattered. It had shown him the strength of his community, the love of his family, and the resilience of the human spirit. And for that, Noah was grateful.

In the eye of the storm, Noah found his calm. He found his strength. He found his hope. And with that, he faced each new day with renewed determination.

As the pandemic raged on, Noah found himself becoming a pillar of strength for his family and his students. His wife, constantly exposed to the virus at the hospital, relied on him for emotional support. His children, confused and scared, looked to him for reassurance. His students, struggling with the abrupt shift to online learning, depended on him for guidance. Noah, in turn, drew strength from them, their resilience and courage inspiring him to keep going.

The pandemic also brought about unexpected changes in Noah's life. He found himself spending more time with his family, their busy schedules replaced by shared meals, movie nights, and long conversations. He discovered new facets of his children's personalities, their unique perspectives on the world around them often leaving him amazed. He found a deeper connection with his wife, their shared experiences bringing them closer than ever before.

In his professional life, Noah found new ways to engage his students, using technology to create interactive lessons and virtual experiments. He found himself learning from his students, their adaptability and creativity in the face of adversity a constant source of inspiration. He also found a new appreciation for his colleagues, their collective efforts to ensure the continuity of education a testament to their dedication and commitment.

As the months passed, Noah watched the world slowly adapt to the new normal. He saw businesses reopening with new safety measures, people venturing out with masks and sanitizers, and communities coming together to support each other. He saw the world healing, slowly but surely.

The pandemic was a storm that had upended Noah's life, but it was also a storm that had brought about unexpected changes. It had forced him to slow down, to reflect, to appreciate the simple joys of life. It had shown him the strength of his community, the resilience of his family, and the adaptability of his students. It had taught him valuable lessons about resilience, adaptability, and the power of hope.

As the year drew to a close, Noah found himself reflecting on the journey he had undertaken. It had been a year of challenges and changes, of fear and uncertainty, but also of growth and learning. He had seen the worst of times, but he had also seen the best of humanity. He had seen people come together in the face of adversity, their collective strength a beacon of hope in the darkest of times.

Noah's life had changed in ways he could never have imagined. He had learned to navigate the storm, to find calm amidst the chaos, to keep going even when the path ahead was uncertain. He had learned to appreciate the simple joys of life, the comfort of a shared meal, the laughter of his children, and the quiet moments with his wife. He had learned to value the power of community, the strength of unity, and the importance of compassion.

As Noah looked ahead to the new year, he did so with a sense of hope and optimism. The storm was not yet over, but he knew that they would weather it together. He knew that they would emerge from it stronger and more resilient. He knew that they would find their way back to normal, a new normal perhaps, but a normal, nonetheless.

The arrival of the pandemic had been a test of Noah's strength, but it had also been a journey of discovery. He had discovered a strength he didn't know he possessed, a resilience he didn't know he had, a hope he didn't know he needed. He had discovered the calm amidst the storm.

CHAPTER 3: INITIAL REACTIONS AND ADJUSTMENTS

When the pandemic hit, Noah's initial reaction was one of shock and disbelief. The news of a global crisis seemed surreal, and he struggled to comprehend the magnitude of the situation and the impact it would have on his daily life. Fear and uncertainty gripped his heart, leaving him wondering what the future held.

As the pandemic continued to unfold, Noah found himself on an emotional rollercoaster. Anxiety, sadness, and frustration became his constant companions. The relentless news updates and the fear of contracting the virus took a toll on his mental health. He yearned for stability and control in such an unpredictable time, but it seemed elusive.

Noah, like many others, had to quickly adjust to working from home. At first, it was a challenge to establish a work-life balance and create a productive workspace within the confines of his home. However, with time, he learned to set boundaries, establish a routine, and make the most of the situation. Remote work became his new normal, and he discovered the joys of flexibility and the absence of a daily commute.

Social isolation weighed heavily on Noah's heart. He missed the warmth of face-to-face interactions with friends and family. Loneliness and isolation became unwelcome guests in his life. To combat this, he started scheduling regular virtual hangouts and game nights, using technology to bridge the physical distance and stay connected with loved ones.

To combat the monotony of being at home, Noah decided to explore new hobbies. He picked up a paintbrush, delved into gardening, and even started learning to play a musical instrument. These activities provided him with a sense of purpose and helped him stay engaged and motivated during the pandemic. The creative outlets became his sanctuary, allowing him to escape the worries of the world, if only for a little while.

Recognizing the importance of mental health, Noah made it a priority to take care of himself. He incorporated mindfulness practices into his daily routine, embracing meditation and yoga to find inner peace amidst the chaos. Additionally, he sought therapy to navigate the emotional challenges brought on by the pandemic. Through therapy, he discovered coping mechanisms and gained valuable insights into his own resilience.

Despite the difficulties, Noah tried to find silver linings in the midst of the pandemic. He appreciated the slower pace of life, the opportunity to spend more time with his immediate family, and the chance to reconnect with old friends virtually. These positive aspects helped him maintain a more optimistic outlook, reminding him that even in the darkest times, there is always a glimmer of hope.

The uncertainty surrounding the pandemic was a constant source of stress for Noah. He had to learn to accept that there were many things beyond his control. Instead of dwelling on the unknown, he focused on taking things one day at a time, finding solace in the present moment. It was a lesson in surrendering to the flow of life and finding peace amidst the chaos.

Noah recognized the importance of seeking support during this challenging time. He reached out to friends, family, and online communities to share his experiences and find comfort in knowing he wasn't alone. Connecting with others who were going through similar struggles provided him with a sense of solidarity and reminded him that we are all in this together.

Over time, Noah developed resilience and grew stronger in the face of adversity. He learned to adapt to the ever-changing circumstances and found strength within himself to navigate the challenges. The pandemic became a catalyst for personal growth, teaching him the importance of resilience and reminding him of the indomitable human spirit. Noah emerged from this experience with a newfound appreciation for life's simple joys and a deeper understanding of his own capacity for strength and growth.

CHAPTER 4: THE DESCENT INTO ISOLATION

As the pandemic tightened its grip In Florida, the state's once-bustling streets fell into an eerie silence. The lockdown, initially a temporary measure, stretched on indefinitely. The virus had forced the world to a standstill, and with it, Noah Thompson found himself descending into a world of isolation.

The first few days were filled with a strange sense of novelty. Noah, like many others, had never experienced anything like this before. The sudden halt of daily routines, the quiet streets, the constant news updates - it all felt surreal. But as the days turned into weeks, the novelty wore off, replaced by a creeping sense of loneliness.

Noah's home, once a place of comfort and warmth, began to feel like a cage. The walls seemed to close in on him, the silence echoing in his ears. His family was his only source of human interaction, their presence a comforting reminder that he was not alone. But even their company couldn't fill the void left by the absence of his students, his colleagues, and his friends.

The isolation was not just physical, but also emotional. Noah found himself grappling with feelings of fear, anxiety, and uncertainty. The constant barrage of news updates, the rising death toll, the uncertainty of the future - it all weighed heavily on his mind. He found himself missing the simple pleasures of life - a shared laugh with a friend, a casual chat with a colleague, a spontaneous trip to the park with his kids.

His work, too, suffered in isolation. Teaching online was a far cry from the interactive, hands-on experience of a physical classroom. Noah missed the energy of his students, the lively discussions, and the shared moments of discovery. The screen, no matter how advanced, could not replicate the human connection that was at the heart of teaching.

Yet, amidst Yet, amidst the isolation, Noah found moments of resilience. He found it in the way his students adapted to online learning, their eagerness to learn undeterred by the circumstances. He found it in the way his family came together, their shared experiences strengthening their bond. He found it in the way his community rallied together, their collective efforts a beacon of hope in these trying times.

Noah also found ways to cope with the isolation. He took up gardening, the act of nurturing plants serving as a therapeutic escape from the harsh reality. He started a virtual book club with his friends, their shared love for literature a comforting reminder of the world outside. He spent more time with his family, their shared meals and movie nights were a source of joy and comfort.

But perhaps the most significant coping mechanism for Noah was his work. Despite the challenges, he found a sense of purpose in teaching. He spent hours preparing lessons, recording videos, and answering emails, his dedication fueled by the desire to provide his students with a sense of normalcy. His work, in many ways, became his lifeline, a constant in the sea of uncertainty.

The descent into isolation was a test of Noah's resilience. It pushed him to his limits, challenging him in ways he had never imagined. But it also revealed a strength he didn't know he possessed. He learned to adapt, to persevere, to find hope in the darkest of times.

As the weeks turned into months, Noah held on to that hope. He held on to the belief that this storm, too, would pass. That they would emerge from it stronger and more resilient. That they would find their way back to normal, a new normal perhaps, but a normal, nonetheless.

The descent into isolation was a journey of self-discovery for Noah. He discovered a strength he didn't know he possessed, a resilience he didn't know he had, a hope he didn't know he needed. He discovered the power.

CHAPTER 5: THE STRUGGLE WITH MENTAL HEALTH BEGINS

As the isolation continued, Noah found himself grappling with a new challenge - his mental health. The constant solitude, the uncertainty of the future, the fear of the unknown - it all began to take a toll on his mind. He found himself slipping into a state of constant worry, his thoughts consumed by the pandemic and its repercussions.

The pandemic was not just a physical health crisis; it was a mental health crisis as well. The isolation, the uncertainty, the fear - it was taking a toll on his mental health. He found himself feeling anxious and restless, his mind filled with negative thoughts and worries. Sleep became elusive, and when it did come, it was often filled with unsettling dreams. He found himself snapping at his family over trivial matters, his patience wearing thin. He felt a constant sense of dread, a feeling that something bad was about to happen.

Noah tried to hide his feelings, to put on a brave face for his family. He didn't want them to worry, to add to their own fears and anxieties. But as the days turned into weeks, and the weeks into months, his mental health continued to deteriorate. He felt like he was on a downward spiral, his mind a whirlpool of negative thoughts and emotions.

He reached out to a therapist, seeking professional help. The sessions were conducted online, a new experience for Noah. He found it difficult to open up, to express his fears and anxieties. But as he continued with the therapy, he started feeling a sense of relief. It was comforting to know that he was not alone and that there were others who were going through the same struggles.

Despite the therapy, Noah's mental health continued to be a struggle. There were good days and bad days, highs and lows. There were days when he felt like he was making progress, and there were days when he felt like he was back to square one. It was a constant battle, a battle that he was determined to win.

As the pandemic raged on, Noah found himself at the edge of his sanity. He was a man pushed to his limits, a man fighting an unseen enemy. His story is a testament to the mental toll of the pandemic, a stark reminder of the unseen battles many are fighting.

Sleep became elusive for Noah. He would lie awake at night, his mind racing with thoughts and fears. The silence of the night seemed to amplify his worries, the darkness a reflection of his state of mind. He would toss and turn, the hours ticking by, until exhaustion finally claimed him.

His appetite, too, began to wane. Meals became a chore, the act of eating a mere necessity rather than a source of enjoyment. He found himself losing interest in things he once loved - his garden lay neglected, his books unread, his guitar untouched.

Noah also began to experience bouts of anxiety. The mere thought of stepping outside, of exposing himself to the virus, would send his heart racing. He found himself constantly checking the news, his anxiety fueled by the rising numbers and grim predictions. His work, once a source of comfort, became a source of stress, the pressure to perform in these trying times overwhelming him.

Depression, too, began to creep in. Noah found himself feeling hopeless, the endless cycle of isolation and fear draining him of his positivity. He found himself withdrawing from his family, his mood swings and irritability straining their relationships. He found himself crying for no apparent reason, the tears a reflection of his inner turmoil.

Recognizing the signs, Noah knew he needed help. He reached out to another therapist, their virtual sessions a lifeline in his struggle. He began to practice mindfulness, the act of focusing on the present moment as a welcome distraction from his worries. He started journaling, the act of penning down his thoughts and fears a therapeutic release. He also started exercising regularly, the physical activity is a natural mood booster.

His family, too, rallied around him. They offered their support and understanding, their love a comforting balm for his troubled mind. They encouraged him to talk about his feelings, their open conversations a step towards breaking the stigma around mental health.

The struggle with mental health was a new battle for Noah. It was a battle fought not in the physical world, but within the confines of his mind. It was a battle that tested his strength and resilience, pushing him to his limits. But it was also a battle that taught him the importance of mental health, the need for self-care, and the power of seeking help.

Despite the challenges, Noah refused to let his mental health define him. He chose to fight, to seek help, to take care of himself. He chose to talk about his struggles, to break the silence around mental health. He chose to hope, to believe in better days.

The struggle with mental health was a journey of self-discovery for Noah. He discovered the importance of mental health, the power of seeking help, and the strength within him. He discovered that it was okay to not be okay, that it was okay to seek help, and that it was okay to take care of himself.

As times pass, Noah continued his battle with mental health. He continued to seek help, practice self-care, and talk about his struggles. He continued to hope, to believe in better days, and to fight.

Noah's journey was not easy. There were days when he felt like giving up, days when the darkness seemed too overwhelming. But he chose to keep going, to keep fighting, to keep believing. He chose to face his fears, to confront his demons, to seek help. He chose to take care of himself, to prioritize his mental health, to practice self-care.

His therapist, too, played a crucial role in his journey. She offered him a safe space to express his feelings, to confront his fears, to seek help. She guided him through his struggles, her expertise and understanding a guiding light in his journey.

As Noah looked back on his journey, he realized that his struggle with mental health was not a weakness, but a testament to his strength. It was a part of his story, a part of who he was. It was a battle he fought and continued to fight, a battle that made him stronger, a battle that made him more resilient.

Noah also realized that his struggle with mental health was not something to be ashamed of. He realized that mental health was just as important as physical health, that it was okay to seek help, that it was okay to take care of himself. He realized that his mental health was a priority, that it was something he needed to take care of, and that it was something he needed to prioritize.

CHAPTER 6: THE DARK DAYS OF DESPAIR

The dark days of despair arrived like an uninvited guest, casting a long, ominous shadow over Noah's life. The world as he knew it seemed to shift, the vibrancy of life replaced by a dull, monotonous grey. The isolation that he had initially embraced as a necessary precaution now felt like a prison, trapping him within the confines of his own home and his own mind.

The fear, once a distant concern, had now become a constant companion. It lurked in the corners of his mind, whispering worst-case scenarios and amplifying his anxieties. The fear of the unknown, the fear of the future, the fear of the virus - it all seemed to converge into a single, overwhelming entity that consumed his thoughts and haunted his dreams.

His constant struggle with his mental health had culminated in a period of profound sadness and hopelessness. The joy and optimism that once defined him seemed to have evaporated, leaving behind a shell of the man he once was. His laughter, once a common sound in the house, had become a rare occurrence, replaced by sighs of frustration and whispers of despair.

His once vibrant world seemed to lose its color, replaced by a monochrome palette of despair. The walls of his home once filled with warmth and love, now seemed cold and distant. The rooms, once bustling with activity, now echoed with silence. The house, once a sanctuary, now felt like a cage. The laughter and joy that once filled his home were replaced by an oppressive silence, punctuated only by his own sobs. The sound of his own voice once filled with enthusiasm and positivity, now carried a note of desolation. The silence was deafening, a constant reminder of his isolation and despair.

His garden, once a sanctuary of peace and tranquility, lay neglected and withered. The flowers that once bloomed in vibrant colors now drooped, their petals falling one by one, mirroring his own state of mind. The once lush green grass was now a dull brown, the life sucked out of it, much like the joy sucked out of his life.

His work, once a source of purpose and fulfillment, became a daunting task. Each lesson felt like a mountain to climb, each assignment a Herculean task. The passion he once had for his work seemed to have evaporated, replaced by a sense of dread and anxiety.

The dark days of despair were a test of Noah's spirit, a battle against his own mind. Each day was a struggle, each moment a fight. The darkness seemed to engulf him, the light at the end of the tunnel growing dimmer with each passing day.

But even in his darkest hours, Noah held on to a glimmer of hope. It was a tiny spark, barely visible amidst the darkness, but it was there. It was this spark that kept him going, that gave him the strength to face each day, to fight his demons, to hold on.

He held on to the belief that these days too shall pass, that brighter days would eventually dawn. He held on to the hope that he would once again find joy, that he would once again laugh, that he would once again find peace. He held on because he knew that this was not the end, but merely a chapter in his life, a chapter that would eventually come to a close.

CHAPTER 7: THE FIGHT FOR SANITY

The fight for sanity was a battle that Noah had never anticipated. It was a battle that was fought not on a physical battlefield, but within the confines of his own mind. It was a battle that was not against an external enemy but against his own thoughts, his own fears, and his own despair.

Each day was a struggle, each moment a test of his strength and resilience. The constant worry, the relentless fear, the overwhelming sadness - it all seemed to converge into a single, formidable adversary that threatened to consume him. But Noah was not one to back down. He was a fighter, and he was determined to reclaim his sanity, to reclaim his life.

He started with small steps. He began to practice mindfulness, focusing on the present moment rather than worrying about the future. He found solace in the simple act of breathing, the rhythmic rise and fall of his chest a reminder that he was alive, that he was here, that he was present.

He also started journaling, penning down his thoughts and fears, hopes, and dreams. The act of writing was therapeutic, a release of the pent-up emotions that threatened to overwhelm him. It was a way for him to confront his fears, face his demons, to make sense of the chaos that seemed to reign within his mind.

Noah also sought professional help. He reached out to two different therapists, their virtual sessions a lifeline in his fight for sanity. The therapists provided him with tools and techniques to manage his anxiety and depression, navigate through the dark days of despair, and find the light amidst the darkness.

Exercise became a crucial part of his routine. He found that physical activity helped to clear his mind, to release the tension that had built up in his body. He started with simple exercises, gradually increasing the intensity as his strength returned. The sweat, the exertion, the feeling of accomplishment after each workout - it all helped to lift his spirits, to give him a sense of control over his life.

He also turned to meditation, finding peace in the silence, in the act of focusing on his breath, on the rhythm of his heartbeat. It was a practice that helped him to center himself, to find a sense of calm amidst the storm that raged within him.

Noah also found solace in nature. He started to tend to his neglected garden, the act of nurturing the plants mirroring his own journey toward healing. The sight of the first bud, the first bloom, filled him with a sense of hope, a reminder that life continues and that there is beauty even in the midst of despair.

He also reconnected with his passion for teaching. He found that helping his students and seeing them grow and learn, gave him a sense of purpose, a sense of fulfillment. It was a reminder of his worth, of his contribution to the world, of his ability to make a difference.

The fight for sanity was not an easy one. There were days when Noah felt like giving up, days when the darkness seemed too overwhelming. But he held on, he persevered, he fought. He fought for his sanity, for his life, for his future.

And slowly, he started to see a change. The darkness started to recede, the light at the end of the tunnel growing brighter. The fear, the anxiety, the despair - they began to lose their grip on him. He found himself laughing more, crying less. He found himself looking forward to each day, rather than dreading it. He found himself living, rather than merely surviving.

The fight for sanity was a journey, a journey that taught Noah about his strength, his resilience, and his capacity to endure. It was a journey that tested him, pushed him to his limits, that showed him the depths of his courage. It was a journey that, despite its challenges, led him toward healing, towards hope, towards a future filled with possibilities. It was a journey that, in the end, helped Noah reclaim his sanity, reclaim his life, and reclaim himself.

CHAPTER 8: SEEKING HELP IN THE MIDST OF CHAOS

In the midst of the chaos that had become his life, Noah realized that he could not fight this battle alone. The weight of his despair, the intensity of his fear, the depth of his sadness - it was all too much for him to bear alone. He needed help, he needed support, he needed guidance.

The first step was acknowledging this need. It was a difficult step, one that required him to confront his pride, his fear of judgment, and his fear of vulnerability. But Noah knew that this was a necessary step, a crucial step in his journey toward healing. And so, he took it. He acknowledged his need for help, he acknowledged his struggle, and he acknowledged his pain.

The next step was reaching out. He reached out to his family, his friends, and his colleagues. He shared his struggles, his fears, and his pain. He let them in, let them see his vulnerability, his despair. It was a difficult step, one that required courage, one that required trust. But it was a step that brought him relief, that brought him comfort, that brought him support.

He also reached out to professionals. He sought the help of therapists, their virtual sessions a lifeline in the midst of the chaos. The therapist provided him with tools and techniques to manage his anxiety, navigate through his despair, and find the light amidst the darkness.

Noah also joined a support group, a community of individuals who were going through similar struggles. The group provided him with a sense of belonging, a sense of understanding, and a sense of solidarity. It was a space where he could share his experiences, his fears, and his victories. It was a space where he could listen to others, learn from their experiences, and draw strength from their resilience.

He also sought help from his doctor, discussing his mental health issues and exploring possible treatment options. The doctor provided him with valuable advice, guiding him toward a path of recovery. Medication was suggested as a possible aid, and after careful consideration, Noah decided to give it a try.

In addition to seeking help from others, Noah also sought help from within. He started reading the Bible and meditating on the words of God. He found solace in the simple act of breathing, the rhythmic rise and fall of his chest a reminder that he was alive, that he was here, that he was present. Finding peace in the silence, in the act of focusing on his breath, on the rhythm of his heartbeat. It was a practice that helped him to center himself, to find a sense of calm amidst the storm that raged within him.

He also found solace in nature. He started to tend to his neglected garden, the act of nurturing the plants mirroring his own journey toward healing. The sight of the first bud, the first bloom, filled him with a sense of hope, a reminder that life continues and that there is beauty even in the midst of chaos.

Seeking help amid chaos was not an easy journey. It required courage, it required vulnerability, it required trust. But it was a journey that brought Noah relief, that brought him support, that brought him hope. It was a journey that showed him that he was not alone, that he was not helpless, that he was not lost. It was a journey that, despite its challenges, led him toward healing, towards hope, towards a future filled with possibilities. It was a journey that, in the end, helped Noah find peace amidst the chaos, find light amidst the darkness, and find himself amidst the despair.

CHAPTER 9: THE ROAD TO RECOVERY

The road to recovery was not a straight path. It was a winding road, filled with twists and turns, ups and downs, victories, and setbacks. But it was a road that Noah was determined to travel, a road that he knew would lead him towards healing, towards hope, towards a future filled with possibilities.

The first step on this road was acceptance. Noah had to accept his situation, accept his struggles, and accept his pain. It was a difficult step, one that required courage, one that required strength. But it was a necessary step, a step that allowed him to acknowledge his reality, to confront his fears, to face his demons.

The next step was seeking help. Noah reached out to his family, his friends, and his colleagues. He sought the help of a therapist, joined a support group, and consulted with his doctor. He learned to lean on others, to share his burdens, and to seek guidance. It was a step that brought him relief, that brought him support, that brought him hope.

Noah started to practice gratitude. He learned to appreciate the small things in life, the simple pleasures that he had often overlooked. He found joy in the warmth of the sun, in the sound of the rain, in the beauty of a blooming flower. He found happiness in the laughter of his students, in the support of his friends, and in the love of his family. It was a practice that helped him to focus on the positive, to find joy amidst the sorrow, to find hope amidst the despair.

Noah also learned the importance of setting boundaries. He learned to say no, to prioritize his needs, to protect his mental health. He learned to take time for himself, to rest, to recharge, to rejuvenate. It was a practice that helped him to maintain his balance, to preserve his energy, to safeguard his sanity.

He also learned to be patient with himself. Recovery was not a race; it was a journey. It was a journey that required time, that required patience, that required perseverance. Noah learned to celebrate his small victories, acknowledge his progress, and be kind to himself.

He also learned to let go. He let go of his guilt, his regrets, his self-blame. He learned to forgive himself, to accept his mistakes, and to learn from his failures. It was a practice that helped him to move forward, to leave the past behind, to focus on the future.

Noah also learned the importance of hope. Hope was the light that guided him through the darkness, the beacon that led him toward recovery. He learned to nurture this hope, to hold onto it, to let it fuel his journey. It was a practice that helped him to stay positive, to stay motivated, to stay strong.

He also learned the power of resilience. He learned that he was stronger than he thought that he could overcome his struggles, and that he could rise above his despair. He learned to draw strength from his experiences, to use his pain as a stepping stone, and to use his struggles as a catalyst for growth.

Noah also learned the importance of self-love. He learned to appreciate himself, value his worth, and celebrate his uniqueness. He learned to love himself, flaws, and all. It was a practice that helped him to build his self-esteem, to boost his confidence, to strengthen his resolve.

He also learned the power of positivity. He learned to focus on the positive, to look for the silver lining, and to find the good in every situation. He learned to cultivate a positive mindset, to foster positive thoughts, to radiate positive energy. It was a practice that helped him to stay optimistic, to stay hopeful, to stay happy.

Noah also learned the importance of community on his road to recovery. His support group became a safe haven, a place where he could share his experiences, his fears, and his victories. It was a place where he could listen to others, learn from their experiences, draw strength from their resilience. It was a place where he felt understood, where he felt accepted, where he felt supported.

He also learned the value of self-expression. He found solace in art, using it as a medium to express his feelings, his thoughts, and his fears. He painted, he sketched, he sculpted. Each piece was a reflection of his journey, a testament to his struggles, and a tribute to his resilience.

Noah also learned the power of faith in Jesus, the prince of peace. He found comfort in his beliefs, and in his spirituality. He prayed he meditated, and he sought solace in his faith. It was a practice that gave him strength, that gave him hope, that gave him peace.

He also learned the importance of balance. He learned to balance his work and his rest, his social life and his solitude, his physical health, and his mental health. He learned to listen to his body, to heed its signals, to respect its needs. It was a practice that helped him to maintain his health, to preserve his energy, to protect his well-being.

Noah also learned the value of perseverance. He learned that recovery was not a linear process, that there would be setbacks, that there would be challenges. But he also learned that he could overcome these obstacles, that he could rise above these setbacks, and that he could continue on his journey. It was a practice that taught him resilience, that taught him determination, that taught him strength.

He also learned the importance of self-awareness. He learned to recognize his triggers, understand his emotions, to manage his reactions. He learned to listen to his thoughts, observe his feelings, and understand his behaviors. It was a practice that helped him to gain control over his mental health, to manage his symptoms, and to prevent relapses.

Noah also learned the power of positivity. He learned to focus on the positive, to look for the silver lining, and to find the good in every situation. He learned to cultivate a positive mindset, to foster positive thoughts, to radiate positive energy. It was a practice that helped him to stay optimistic, to stay hopeful, to stay happy.

He also learned the value of self-compassion. He learned to be kind to himself, to forgive himself, to love himself. He learned to treat himself with the same compassion that he would treat a friend and to speak to himself with the same kindness that he would speak to a loved one. It was a practice that helped him to heal, to grow, to thrive.

Noah also learned the importance of routine. He found comfort in the predictability of a routine, in the stability of a schedule. He learned to structure his day, plan his activities, to manage his time. It was a practice that helped him to stay organized, to stay focused, to stay productive.

He also learned the value of connection. He learned to connect with others, to share his experiences, and to seek support. He learned to connect with himself, to understand his needs, and to honor his feelings. It was a practice that helped him to feel understood, to feel accepted, to feel loved.

CHAPTER 10: LESSONS LEARNED AND THE NEW NORMAL

Throughout the pre- and post-pandemic period, Noah learns several valuable lessons that shape his perspective and approach to life. Here are some of the lessons he discovers:

1. The importance of adaptability: Noah realizes that life is full of unexpected twists and turns. The pandemic serves as a stark reminder that being adaptable and open to change is crucial for navigating challenging times.

2. The significance of human connection: The period of social isolation highlights the deep longing for human connection within Noah. He learns to cherish and nurture his relationships, understanding that genuine connections are essential for emotional well-being.

3. The value of self-care: Noah recognizes the importance of prioritizing his own well-being. He learns that taking care of himself physically, mentally, and emotionally is not selfish but necessary for his overall happiness and resilience.

4. The power of gratitude: The pandemic prompts Noah to reflect on the blessings in his life. He learns to appreciate the little things, finding gratitude in moments of simplicity and recognizing the abundance that surrounds him.

5. The need for resilience: Noah witnesses firsthand the power of resilience in the face of adversity. He learns that setbacks and challenges are opportunities for growth and that resilience is a key trait to cultivate in order to overcome obstacles.

6. The significance of community support: Noah discovers the strength that lies in coming together as a community. He learns the importance of supporting and uplifting one another, realizing that collective efforts can make a significant impact during difficult times.

7. The value of mindfulness and living in the present: The pandemic teaches Noah the importance of living in the present moment. He learns to let go of worries about the future and regrets from the past, finding peace and contentment by fully immersing himself in the present.

8. The impact of personal responsibility: Noah understands that his actions have consequences not only for himself but also for the wider community. He learns the importance of taking personal responsibility for his choices and behaviors, recognizing that they can have a significant impact on the well-being of others.

9. The significance of resilience in uncertainty: The pandemic exposes Noah to a great deal of uncertainty. He learns to embrace the unknown and find strength in navigating through uncertain times, understanding that resilience is a valuable asset in maintaining a positive mindset.

10. The appreciation for the simple joys in life: Through the challenges of the pandemic, Noah gains a newfound appreciation for the simple joys in life. He learns to find happiness in the small moments, realizing that true fulfillment comes from within and can be found even in the most challenging circumstances.

CONCLUSION: A JOURNEY THROUGH MADNESS AND BACK

As we close the pages of "From Sanity to Madness: How the Pandemic Pushed One Man to the Edge of Insanity!", we are left with a profound understanding of the human spirit's resilience. Noah's journey from the brink of despair back to a life of hope and healing is a testament to the strength that lies within us all. His story serves as a stark reminder of the mental health crisis that the pandemic has exacerbated, but it also shines a light on the path to recovery and the importance of seeking help.

Noah's story is not just a tale of survival, but also a narrative of transformation. The lessons he learned along the way, the strength he discovered within himself, and the new normal he embraced, all serve as a beacon of hope for those who find themselves in similar situations. His journey underscores the importance of self-care, resilience, patience, acceptance, positivity, community, self-expression, self-compassion, gratitude, setting boundaries, mindfulness, and forgiveness in the face of adversity.

The pandemic has undeniably pushed many to the edge, but Noah's story is a testament to the fact that it is possible to pull back, find solid ground again, and rebuild a life worth living. His journey serves as a powerful reminder that even in our darkest moments, we are not alone. There is always help available, and there is always hope.

In the end, "From Sanity to Madness: How the Pandemic Pushed One Man to the Edge of Insanity!" is more than just a chronicle of one man's descent into and ascent from madness. It is a call to action, a plea for greater understanding and compassion towards those battling mental health issues, particularly in these unprecedented times. It is a rallying cry for the DE stigmatization of mental health and a push for more accessible mental health resources.

As we reflect on Noah's journey, we are reminded of the importance of maintaining our mental health, reaching out when we need help, and extending a helping hand to those who are struggling. We are reminded that it's okay not to be okay and that seeking help is not a sign of weakness, but of strength. Above all, we are reminded of the power of the human spirit to overcome even the most formidable challenges. Noah's story is a testament to the resilience inherent in us all, a beacon of hope in the face of adversity, and a powerful reminder that even in the midst of a pandemic, we can find our way back to sanity.

EPILOGUE: LIFE AFTER THE PANDEMIC

As we step into the aftermath of Noah's journey, we find ourselves in a world forever changed by the pandemic. Yet, amidst the chaos and uncertainty, there is a glimmer of hope. Noah's story, his descent into madness, and his subsequent rise to sanity serve as a beacon of light in these dark times. His resilience, his strength, and his unwavering spirit are a testament to the indomitable human will to survive and thrive, even in the face of adversity.

Noah's transformation is not just a personal victory, but a symbol of hope for all those grappling with mental health issues. His story underscores the importance of seeking help, acknowledging our struggles, and embracing our vulnerabilities. It reminds us that it's okay to not be okay, that it's okay to ask for help, and that it's okay to take time to heal. It reassures us that even in our darkest moments, we are not alone.

In the wake of the pandemic, Noah's journey serves as a call to action. It urges us to destigmatize mental health, foster a culture of understanding and compassion, and make mental health resources more accessible. It implores us to reach out to those who are struggling, to lend a listening ear, and to extend a helping hand. It encourages us to be kind, not just to others, but also to ourselves.

As we navigate our way through this new normal, Noah's story serves as a guide. It teaches us the importance of self-care, resilience, patience, acceptance, positivity, community, self-expression, self-compassion, gratitude, setting boundaries, mindfulness, and forgiveness. It reminds us that these are not just buzzwords, but essential tools for maintaining our mental health and well-being.

 As we close this chapter and look toward the future, we carry with us the lessons from Noah's journey. We are reminded of the strength that lies within each of us, the resilience that we are capable of, and the hope that can be found even in the darkest of times. We are inspired by Noah's transformation, his courage, and his unwavering spirit. We are moved by his story, his struggles, and his triumphs.

Noah's journey from sanity to madness and back again is a testament to the human spirit's resilience. It is a story of hope, of healing, and of the power of the human will. It is a story that resonates with us all, a story that inspires us, a story that gives us hope.

As we move forward, we do so with a renewed sense of purpose, a heightened awareness of the importance of mental health, and a deep appreciation for the strength and resilience of the human spirit. We carry with us the lessons we have learned, the inspiration we have drawn, and the hope we have found in Noah's story.

In the end, "From Sanity to Madness: How the Pandemic Pushed One Man to the Edge of Insanity!" is not just Noah's story, but our story too. It is a story of resilience, of hope, and of the power of the human spirit. It is a story that reminds us that even in the face of adversity, we can find our way back to sanity.

RESOURCES FOR MENTAL HEALTH SUPPORT

1. National Alliance on Mental Illness (NAMI): NAMI provides information, resources, and support for individuals and families affected by mental health conditions. They offer helplines, support groups, educational programs, and advocacy initiatives. Visit their website at www.nami.org.

2. Mental Health America (MHA): MHA is a leading community-based nonprofit organization dedicated to promoting mental health and preventing mental illness. They offer screening tools, educational resources, and a variety of support programs. Visit their website at www.mhanational.org.

3. Crisis Text Line: Crisis Text Line provides free, 24/7 support for individuals in crisis. Text "HOME" to 741741 to connect with a trained crisis counselor. Visit their website at www.crisistextline.org.

4. Substance Abuse and Mental Health Services Administration (SAMHSA): SAMHSA is a government agency that provides resources and support for mental health and substance abuse issues. They offer a national helpline, treatment locator, and various educational materials. Visit their website at www.samhsa.gov.

5. American Psychological Association (APA): The APA offers resources for finding psychologists, understanding different mental health conditions, and accessing evidence-based treatments. Visit their website at www.apa.org.

6. Therapy for Black Girls: Therapy for Black Girls is an online directory that connects Black women and girls with mental health professionals who specialize in serving their needs. They also provide a podcast and other resources. Visit their website at www.therapyforblackgirls.com.

7. LGBTQ+ National Help Center: The LGBTQ+ National Help Center provides support, resources, and a helpline specifically for LGBTQ+ individuals. Visit their website at www.glbthotline.org.

8. Veterans Crisis Line: The Veterans Crisis Line offers free, confidential support for veterans in crisis and their families. Call 1-800-273-8255 and press 1, or text 838255 to connect with a trained responder. Visit their website at www.veteranscrisisline.net.

9. Online Therapy Platforms: Platforms like BetterHelp, Talkspace, and Amwell offer online therapy services, allowing individuals to connect with licensed therapists through video, phone, or chat sessions. These platforms often provide affordable and convenient options for mental health support.

10. Local Mental Health Organizations: Check with your local community centers, hospitals, or mental health clinics for resources and support groups available in your area. They may offer counseling services, support groups, or referrals to other mental health professionals.